Faith Defeated
My Pain

A Short Story of a Soul who Defeated Cancer

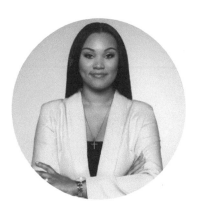

By: Jasmine J. Pettross

Foreword by Dr. Tamika S. Hood

Faith Defeated my Pain: A Short Story of a Soul who Defeated Cancer

Requests for information should be addressed to:
Jasmine J. Pettross
jasminenae510@yahoo.com

ISBN 978-1-7346599-2-4

Cover design: Perfect_designx
Interior design: Aalishaa
Printed in the United States of America

Contents

Dedication

This book honors me and everyone who has survived or succumbed to cancer or lost a loved one from the illness.

Acknowledgments

First and foremost, I give all thanks to God for His blessings that he has showered upon me and His patience with me throughout this process. Thank you for giving me the ability to share my testimony with others and giving me strength throughout my life. One day, I heard this little voice in my head after my diagnosis; I knew it was You. "Jasmine, you are going to write a book." You have always believed in me, and I am forever grateful for your love. You are truly my savior.

Thank you to my treatment team because I would not be here without you all as well! I'm so thankful for my surgeon and for performing successful surgeries during my journey. I can't thank you enough! The removal of my tumor was one of the best days of my life and I am beyond grateful for your care and ability to remove my cancer.

To my Fiancé, the moment we met in the same apartment building, you have always been very supportive. Thank you for praying with me, loving, and pushing me to continue writing my story. Your drive makes me drive even harder. You inspire me to get up each day and live in my purpose. I am eternally grateful to have you in my life. I love you!

Mom, thank you for being supportive and having my back through it all! I will forever be grateful for everything you do and for guiding me through life. Thank you for the sacrifices that you have made, the lessons you have taught, and your unconditional love! You are appreciated, and you deserve your roses! I love you!

Dad, (King Don), thank you for your understanding/ humor and for being there when I need to vent. Thanks for motivating and encouraging me to keep pushing at my lowest points in life! You always know how to put a smile on my face by being you! You have a special place in my heart. I love you!

Desmond, you are an Angel, and you are my brother! Thank you for never judging me and being supportive of my dreams. You are the most positive person; believe it or not, you keep me sane and make me want to work harder! I love you!

Thank you to my 2nd parents, my grandparents. Nana and Dar, thank you for molding me into the person I am today. I will be forever grateful for the love and guidance you give each day. You both are my heart! I love you.

To my editor, publisher, and friend Dr. Tamika S. Hood, I would like to thank you for believing in me and helping me with this overall process. You have been a great listener, and I appreciate your making my vision come to light. It has been some challenging days, but you were always there to keep my spirit going, provided me with motivational tips to believe in myself, and prayed with me numerous times! You are one of the strongest women. I can't thank you enough! I love you!

Many thanks to my friends for uplifting me through these trying times. You know who you are, and I thank God for bringing each of you into my life! To my family on both sides- aunts, uncles, cousins, and family friends- thank you for your thoughtfulness and support throughout the journey! From the gifts, talks on the phone, and overall being there for me! I cannot thank you enough! I love you all!

Thank you to my prayer warriors for all your prayers and advice thus far! I also want to thank my readers! Thank you for taking the time out of your day to read my testimony. I hope it gives you inspiration and a different outlook on life!

Foreword

There is power and purpose in pain. The Word says that "weeping may endure for a night, but joy comes in the morning" Psalm 30:5 (NKJV). As a Professional Certified Coach, college professor, motivational speaker, author, publisher, and industrial-organizational psychologist-practitioner, I have helped clients navigate the nuances of unpacking their pain. Jasmine J. Pettross exemplifies power personified by the purpose in her pain. As Jasmine tells her sensational story of surviving cancer at a young age, you will be inspired by her strength and positivity. She leans on God's Word to carry her through her storm.

In my book Out of the Wilderness: Weathering Life's Storms from Trials Through Triumph, I use poetry and prose to describe how weathering the storms of life can make you weary. Yet when you cast your cares on God, He will give you the strength you need not only to survive but thrive. And thriving is what Jasmine is doing. Even though she has triumphed over her storm, she desires to be a blessing to others who can learn from her experience.

As you read this monumentally motivational book, open your heart, and let God speak to you through Jasmine's tantalizing testimony. There is a place for you to write your self-reflections and even a Q&A section and pictures of Jasmine's journey. Jasmine J. Pettross inspires me with her optimism in the face of adversity. She does not look like what she has been through. Her heart is huge, and her smile is energizing. Jasmine was my strength when I was at one of my lowest points, suffering from anxiety and depression. I will never forget years ago when she visited me when I did not want to get out of bed or see people. She was persistent as she waited downstairs for hours until I finally came out of my room. Tears poured from my eyes as she told me her story, which resonated with me. Her optimism and openness to share her experiences and resources with me is something I will always cherish, as she is such a supportive friend. I love her and her strong spirit, and you will, too.

This brilliant book reveals resilience through the highs and lows of life that Jasmine has faced. Some parts of her sentimental story will make you cry, and others will bring a smile to your face and joy to your heart. Jasmine's story is not only about cancer; it is about faith. Faith to believe that God will defeat your dragons, whatever they may be. For some, it's cancer. For others, it's the pain of losing someone. And for most, it's getting back up when life knocks you down. As I wrote in Out of the Wilderness, "God is greater than it all. Once you increase your faith and hand your situation over to God, He will guide your path and lead you to deliverance."

This "Short Story of a Soul who Defeated Cancer" is poignant and powerful. So, get ready to join Jasmine on this journey of faith that defeated her pain!

Introduction

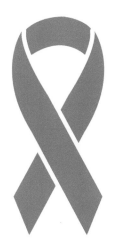

The purpose of this short story is to share my testimony and to inform readers of difficult situations that could be encountered in life. Imagine how the ending results of a long battle build a person's strength and how having faith is the ultimate road to advancement in life.

There is a purpose in life that comes in the form of pain, but this book defines the meaning of perseverance. My faith in God saved my life and will now help me save others. This short story is broken into three parts that detail the beginning through the outcome of my journey.

"Bless the Lord O my soul and forget not all His benefits; Who forgives all your iniquities, Who heals all your diseases." Psalm 103:2-3 (NKJV)

This book will introduce you to raw evidence that God is real and merciful in all ways. Readers will grasp the concept of the three major roles that played a part in my journey, Living With Purpose, From Pain to Promotion, and My Pain converted into Blessings. Each one signifies the events of the trauma and reality that were faced through this process.

Along with motivational touches and inspirational segments, this story will also touch on self-reflection topics, plus a Q&A section that will give you more context of Jasmine's journey.

Sit back and read the powerful story of a woman that has faced a life-threatening illness but learned about her reason for living while on the journey.

> **As soon as I gave myself to God, the blessings started coming.**

Living With Purpose

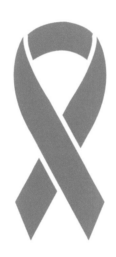

What if you woke up one day and your world turned upside down? What if the only way you could have kids was by freezing your eggs because you may not be able to carry the baby? What if you woke up and had to take a drug every day that made you sick to your stomach while also going through multiple surgeries and having needles stuck into you every day? What if you had to get radiation treatment, and the end results involved constant pain? Things can be taken from you instantly, but life has its way of changing you. God has his way of changing a person. He also has his way of being on time. He gives second chances, and he shows up. He saves lives. He is alive. He saved my life.

For a long time, I was feeling weak and cramping in my stomach, along with seeing blood in my stool. I did not think it was anything consequential and thought I was cramping because I was about to come on my menstrual cycle.

After a while, I knew something was going on with my body because every time I had a bowel movement, I would see a fair amount of blood coming from my anus. I also felt fatigued and assumed it was from working long shifts. I worked at a mental hospital for a while and thought I was constantly drained because I had to work late nights. I told the doctors my symptoms. They gave me a stool kit that examines your stool for bacteria, viruses, or other germs. I went to pick up the stool kit and sat it down in my room because I did not have the time to administer it yet.

A year passed, and my mom, brother, and I moved, so the stool kit was misplaced. Months went by, and I still had the same symptoms; honestly, life got in the way. I ended up getting a new job working with kids, and I was constantly drained and felt abdominal cramping. At the end of February 2016, I was at work and stepped out to use the bathroom because I was in excruciating pain. I noticed that I was bleeding from my rectum. I was devastated. I then knew something was wrong. I was terrified because I knew I was going on vacation soon. I was about to go on a cruise the next month to the Bahamas.

I had planned for this trip six months in advance. As I needed to take care of this matter asap, I went to the doctors again, and they gave me another stool kit. I finished the stool kit and returned it to the lab for diagnosis. I waited a few days to hear my results. The results returned positive for blood in my stool, and the doctor who provided me with the kit referred me to a gastroenterologist (gastro) specialist. I walked out of the doctor's office frustrated because I already knew there was blood in my stool, to begin with, and the process was lingering to find out what was going on with me.

Meanwhile, I had some shopping to do for my trip! All I could think about was this mini-break because I needed a vacation! A day after my appointment, I scheduled another one with the gastro specialist to follow up. I wanted to get the appointment out of the way before I traveled. I had to wait a few weeks before seeing the doctor. A few weeks passed, and it was time for my appointment. The gastro specialist asked me multiple questions regarding my symptoms and family history. I really did not want to tell her how long I had the symptoms. I took a deep breath and said, "one year" (Sigh). She was shocked and said, "Wow, why did you wait that long?" I proceeded to tell her I thought it was nothing. She began talking to me about the next steps and said she wanted to schedule me for a colonoscopy to better look at my colon and rectum.

I had no idea what a colonoscopy was, so I did not know what to expect. The gastro specialist told me many people don't get colonoscopies until they are in their 50s, but I was an exception. She said it would be a minor procedure, and I would be given anesthesia to put me to sleep. I was distressed because God knows I hate needles and to be put to sleep. I would have to get an IV in my arm! I cried all day. She also said I would have to drink a prep called Golytely and fast for a day or two. I'm not the best with unpleasant drinks, but she voiced that the drink does a better job cleaning out your system, and a pill wouldn't be as effective. I was informed of the importance of ensuring I drank the whole bottle. It was important for my system to be cleaned out so they could see everything inside. After I was instructed with this information, I scheduled my colonoscopy to be done after I returned from my trip.

When I got home from my meeting with the doctor, all I could think about was my trip. I told myself I would have all the fun I could because I had to go through that procedure when I returned. A few days later, as I was packing, I started having bad cramping in my stomach. I looked at my calendar, and it wasn't time for my menstrual. I was baffled. That moment, I realized I had been having cramps for almost a year and brushed it off like it was nothing! I took a deep breath, sat down on the bed, and thought, "Wow," something is really not right.

When my mom came home that evening, I told her that I was having cramps, and she suggested getting my colonoscopy before I went on my trip. I did not want to do that because I wanted something to look forward to before proceeding with the colonoscopy. I told myself I would get the procedure done so I could get it out of the way, and then I would not have to worry about getting it done after the trip. The following day, I called to schedule a colonoscopy, and they gave me an appointment for the following week.

Time went by, and it was the day before my procedure. I dreaded this day because I knew the prep would be horrible! I read some reviews about having a colonoscopy procedure, and most people said the prep is the hardest part. I had to begin to fast the whole day and be on a clear, liquid diet. I could have popsicles, drinks, chicken broth, etc. I had to make sure the color of the items was not red. I was starving that day. Everyone knows that if I do not eat, I get angry! The worst part about that day was drinking the prep "Golytely." I had to mix the drink with water and drink the whole 64-ounce jug. I was up all night crying while trying to down the drink. I started consuming it at 5 p.m. that day and did not end the prep until 2 a.m.

I called the doctors that day and begged them for pills to clean me out, but they told me pills would not clean me out. They insisted that I be strong and drink it. I thought, "you do not know what it's like to drink this; it just isn't fair!" I called my aunts on my mom's side, and they insisted I suck it up and stop acting like a coward. I was getting mad with everyone because they were not in my shoes. I called my grandmother and grandfather in Florida and my grandmother in Ohio, and they gave me some words of wisdom. They said if you want to find out what is wrong with you, you will drink the drink and do what is best for your health. My mom and I did not see eye to eye the whole time I consumed the drink because I would not listen to her and told her I had given up. She was mad at me because I did not even drink half the bottle, and it was already 10 p.m. She said, "I took off for you tomorrow to help you get to your appointment and to be there for you, and you can't even drink the drink." It sounded good, but I told her I'd just do it when I returned from my cruise! I was not going for it! She kept saying," if you want to keep cramping and keep having blood in your stool, then don't drink it. I care about you and want the best for you."

I went into my room and said a prayer asking God to give me the strength to get the drink down and to numb my taste buds from tasting the drink. I started gulping it down, and finally, after two hours, it was finished. It was 2 a.m. by that time, and I had three hours to sleep until it was time for my procedure, but it was hard because I was in the bathroom all night having bowel movements. Finally, my stool became water, telling me I was clean.

I showered, dressed, and headed to the doctor the following day. The doctor asked me how the prep went, and I frowned. I did not even want to discuss anything about the prep. Before the procedure started, I had to urinate in a cup to ensure I was not pregnant. The nurse advised me to put on a hospital gown and to get comfortable until the technician was ready to stick the IV into my arm. Again, I have always been afraid of needles, so my anxiety began to get extreme. The tech finally came and stuck me; of course, I screamed! My family has always called me a "drama queen," but I did not care!

Once I was done getting prepped for my procedure, a staff member brought my mom into the room, and the doctors came in with documents that needed my signature. Once I signed the forms, I was off to get my procedure done. When I got into the operating room, I started talking to the staff, and then suddenly, I woke up in the recovery room. I thought to myself, I do not even remember falling asleep! I looked to my left, and my mom was right beside me, smiling! She said, "How do you feel?" I answered, "I'm OK." We waited about 10 minutes before the doctor shared the results. I was so happy that it was over; I told myself I never wanted to go through that prep again. Although, the procedure was a piece of cake. The doctor finally came in and asked us if cancer had run in the family. I looked at my mom, shocked, and said, "Um, not that I know of." My mom looked so distraught.

The doctor said it was a 50/50 chance that I had developed cancer because she found a tumor the size of a peach on my rectum. She then said it could be colon cancer. The whole time, I was numb everywhere. I had no emotions. She said she sent it in for a biopsy and told us we should receive the results soon. My mom and I left the doctor's suite. There was silence when we walked onto the elevator. My mom was not talking the whole car ride home. She seemed very troubled. I was not as sad as she was because I did not believe it was cancer. I figured the nurse would phone me to prescribe medicine, and the situation would disappear. Honestly, at that time, I was glad that the procedure was over and that I could continue packing for my trip.

A week passed, and while at work, I received a phone call from the doctor's office. I figured I would forward the call to my answering machine because I was busy. Once I could take a break, I could step out and listen to the message. The message stated, "I'm calling from Johns Hopkins to let you know that your biopsy has come back cancerous, and I would like to schedule an appointment for you to meet with the cancer treatment team at Johns Hopkins Hospital in Baltimore." I could not believe it. I hung up immediately. I said, "I've never heard my heartbeat like this ever." I could not hold the tears back, so I started walking to my director's office and asked if she could talk so that I could vent. Once I walked into her office, I started crying. She was there to confide. After about five minutes, I calmed down and began to tell her the news. She told me that she was there for me and that if there was anything she could do, do not hesitate to ask. After I left her office, I called my mom, and she picked up the phone and said, "I already know." I paused for a moment because I could hear in her voice that she was upset. She also mentioned that I might not be able to go on my trip. I started weeping and questioning why she came up with that observation. She said, "Jasmine, you will have to see; your health is way more important."

When I got home from work, my mom was lying on the couch and had few words to say. I believe sleeping and lying around was how she coped. I started telling my family and friends the news, and everyone was astounded. I told my friend with whom I was going on the trip that there was a chance I would not be able to go, but I would let her know soon. She understood that my health was more crucial. I needed a lot of support. My dad was in town and offered to come with me to some of my appointments, which felt good.

The first week of March 2016, I went to Johns Hopkins with my mom, dad, and brother to talk with my treatment team. I met with the surgeon, nurse, radiation oncologist, and chemo doctor. It was a very long day, and extremely hard to take everything in for all of us. They spoke with me about my cancer and told me it was called Colorectal Cancer and staged it at 3. They went on to say that it was very rare for my age. Many of them were in shock and said I was one of the youngest patients they were dealing with at that time. I was only 23 and going on 24 as of May 2016. The treatment team was very sympathetic and said they would do whatever they could to remove the cancer; I just needed to follow their directions. I asked the doctors if I was going to die. I noticed that they never gave me an exact answer. They expressed that my stage

3 cancer could be cured if they acted quickly and aggressively. They warned me that the process and everything I would have to go through might sound overwhelming, but it is the protocol to provide this information. I had no idea what information they needed to tell me, but I was calm and numbed.

They told me I would have to do some chemo, and after the surgeon removed my cancer, I would have to get back on chemo for some time. The team explained the effects of chemo. They said it could make me nauseous/vomiting, have different taste buds, feel weak and sleepy, have hair loss, and may cause my red blood cells to be low. They said that I would have radiation every day for about six weeks, and I would have to ensure my bladder was full before going for treatment. They indicated that drinking enough water was a must. They then announced that after a few weeks of radiation, I might feel tired and have soreness in my bottom, making it difficult for me to go to the restroom. Yet, they did say that there were ways to help with the pain. They insisted that I did not panic. Another major part of the process was that I might not be able to have children on my own. They recommended that I freeze my eggs. They also communicated that the radiation would hit the lower section of my body, so if I tried to use my eggs, they could be bad eggs, and the team suggested that I not risk that. The doctors said I would have to schedule an appointment with a fertility doctor as soon as possible to get the procedure done because it had to be done before proceeding with radiation. I asked the doctors would the fertility procedure hurt, and they said I would have to discuss that matter with the fertility doctors. Honestly, I'd had enough information for that day. I soon told my parents that I needed some air.

It was getting very overwhelming; I started to cry. Once I had walked back into the room, the doctor told me they were sorry and understood my frustration. The doctor also added that after my surgery, I would be getting a part of my colon taken out and would have to wear an ileostomy bag on my stomach for a year. Sometimes depending on the surgery, it could be permanent. I fell out of my chair; I never thought my life would be like this. I know they say you should never question God, but I asked God why! My mom, dad, and brother looked so sad that it made me feel worse. After the doctors discussed everything, I took a deep breath and said," Will I still be able to go on my trip in a week"? Four doctors responded yes, and one said no. My radiation oncologist suggested I do everything right away. He said, "You don't know if your tumor will grow more during that time and that it might be too late to fix because, at this point, you're stage three, and it's so close to breaking through your wall."

My cancer at this point did not spread, thank God, but going on that trip, who knows if it could have. I respected his honesty but was very disturbed. My family suggested that I get everything I needed to get done and travel later. I told my friend the unpleasant news, and she explained that she understood and that I should do what was best for my health. She said that she was going to keep me in her prayers.

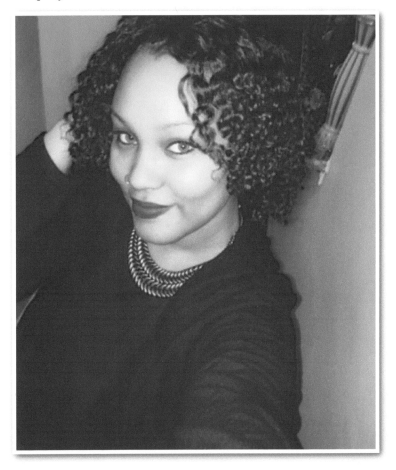

Self-Reflection

What is your purpose? What makes you want to get up each day? What inspires you?

Self-Reflection

Self-Reflection

Self-Reflection

_____

_____

_____

_____

_____

_____

_____

_____

_____

_____

_____

Self-Reflection

Self-Reflection

Self-Reflection

From Pain to Promotions

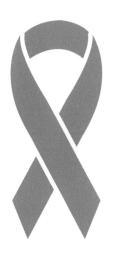

The following week came, and I had to attend my appointment with the fertility doctor. She wanted to start the process for me to get my eggs frozen. She explained the importance of this first step because they had to freeze my eggs before they started the radiation. The treatment team did not want to risk me not having kids. The doctor then explained that I had to get shots in my stomach weekly to retrieve them. Lastly, she explained that they would remove one of my ovaries and move the other out of the way. This is because they did not want my ovaries to be in the way of the radiation. They also would be removing both of my fallopian tubes.

Again, I asked, "Why me." This action plan happened from March 9, 2016, to March 28, 2016. My nurse suggested that I get a cream to numb the areas on my body where I had to get a shot. I could not believe they had a cream; no one had ever suggested that! The cream that the doctor prescribed was called lidocaine. Moving forward, this was a numbing cream I used every time I knew I had to get a shot. In my mind, I thought this was too easy. I just knew the ointment would not be strong enough to work.

The first day I got an injection in my stomach, I used the cream. I put a dab of the cream in the area where I had to get a shot and then covered it with a bandage for at least 30 minutes, as instructed so that it would numb the area. "Wow, that was not bad," I said. For two weeks, I continued to get shots in my abdomen. I went home that night and said a prayer to God. "God, this has been a long crazy month so far. I asked myself, why is this happening to me? What are you trying to prove to me? What are you trying to make me see? Am I going to find purpose in this?" I started screaming. I could not hold the tears in any longer. "I'm letting you know now; I will be strong. I am more than my cancer! I am going to fight and fight until I cannot stop fighting anymore. I am worthy, and I am indestructible. My purpose is deeper. I feel it. God, please give me the strength to make it through. Keep me alive and able to see my future. I'm giving you me, I'm putting everything in your hands, and I'm trusting you."

As soon as I gave myself to God, the blessings started to come in. I felt like the same person but with a different spirit. I started to realize that I needed to take it day by day and not think about the future but think about the present. I had my procedure the following week, and the doctor said, "I retrieved 16 eggs." It was a happy feeling to know that I could still have kids, maybe not on my own, but I would have to find a surrogate. I never in life thought I would freeze my eggs, but God always throws curveballs when we least expect it. The way that I wanted my life, God said no! He wanted it a different way. I needed to adjust to what I had to go through and enjoy life differently. I knew that I would have to sacrifice a lot, especially everything I was used to doing. I had to cut back on alcohol for a year while undergoing chemo and radiation. Now, I'm not going to say that was hard, but sometimes when I wanted to go out with my friends, I could not engage in drinking and would be the quietest one while everyone was taking shots back. Honestly, not drinking wasn't that bad. It was not like I drank a lot. I just loved me some wine! I got accustomed to it and still hung out and enjoyed myself without it!

In April 2016, I was surprised by a visit from my grandparents, who came up from Florida. My mother had called them and asked if they would come to assist in taking me to my treatments. They also made sure I was fed and kept comfortable every day. On April 14, 2016, I began chemotherapy and radiation treatments five days a week (Monday through Friday) for 29 days. Friends and other family members, from time to time, took me to my radiation appointments to relieve my grandparents of having to take me for treatments every day. I felt like the illness had taken over my life. I could only go out and enjoy the fresh air when I was feeling good because sometimes I would feel nauseous and weak. I was on chemo pills. These pills did not make me lose my hair, but they thinned out my hair and eyebrows. The chemo made my hands and feet very dark, and it was hard to get used to the changes my body was going through. I napped a lot because cancer took my energy. Some days I would cut back on foods I usually eat because the taste was not the same. I would eat bananas almost every day but got sick while eating them on most days. I would regurgitate on the days that I felt nauseous. Those were the days I would be close to my bed.

A friend suggested getting motion sickness wristbands that relieve nausea and vomiting. I started wearing those wristbands faithfully; they helped tremendously. Radiation was even worse. Each morning I would have to drink two 32-ounce bottles of water until my bladder was full. I had to go to the bathroom every morning, but I could only empty my bladder once my radiation was finished. The radiation process took about 20 minutes or so each day. The technicians had to ensure they gave me the proper dosage, so they took more time aligning my body on the machine correctly.

I will never forget my radiation experience because I had the best techs! They made my experience almost easy. They let me listen to my favorite songs while I was having my treatments and were always friendly. These treatments felt like a full-time job, so it was nice to have a great support system during this process. After weeks of radiation, things began to take a turn for the worst. I would scream so loud while using the restroom. My anus began to shrink due to the radiation I received daily. The doctor prescribed Aloe Vera gel to help soothe the area, which relieved the pain for the most part. They also recommended that I try a sitz bath. They explained that it would help soothe the irritation. I never had pain while using the bathroom, so this experience was not easy for me.

The month of May came. I was so excited because I knew I would be done with taking chemo orally. I also rang the bell on my last day of radiation! The bell symbolizes an ending to radiation/chemotherapy treatment. Cancer patients often ring a ceremonial bell to acknowledge the end of their treatment. The whole treatment team and other cancer patients gathered around to help celebrate. That day was one of the happiest days of my life. I did not think I would ever go through chemo or radiation in this lifetime. I rang that bell with passion and cried tears of joy that night. I thought to myself, "all those long days and nights trying to get through that horrible medicine that was given to me and that made me sick at times, "Wow, I got through it!" I even faced pain in my bottom every time I had a bowel movement, which felt like I was pooping out knives. It was the most excruciating pain. Those were the moments I felt like God was showing me what my purpose was. On my good days, I stepped out to get fresh air, and some of my friends and family would visit, and I could converse with them.

By this time, it was summer; every June, my friends and I always tried to see my friend's mom on June 16. That was the day my friend passed years ago. That day was an emotional day for me. I sat and talked to her mom and family. It is always enjoyable being around them. Her family always felt like a second family to me. When I discovered I had cancer, I thought, "My friend would not want me to be upset; she was the person who would always encourage me to do more, to do better." Her mom is one of the sweetest people I know. She always gave me such encouraging words, letting me know things would be fine and always sending me positive energies. Even though I had cancer, I was happy to be still able to celebrate my friend's life. After being over there and being around so many beautiful souls, I realized I wanted to share my journey with the world. I wanted to let others know what I was facing because I never knew whom I might help or inspire. Also, many people wanted to keep track of my progress. I had contacts who said, "Wow, I can't believe you're going through this at such a young age." People always felt bad for me. I still could not believe I was going through something like this. Honestly, I wouldn't think about it until someone brought it up, but I gave them words of wisdom because my spirit was too powerful for the sympathy cards given to me.

> "Trust in the LORD with all your heart, And lean not on your own understanding; In all your ways acknowledge Him, And He shall direct your paths."
> Proverbs 3:5-6 (NKJV)

Lord knew I needed a vacation away from home. My best friend mentioned that she and her family were going to Pensacola, Florida, to visit her sister and other family members. I was excited when she asked me if I wanted to go. I told her I would have to get back with her because, at that time, I was under the care of my doctor. The next few days, I sat at home thinking about the opportunity and prayed to God that my doctors would tell me it was OK that I go. I went to my next checkup appointment, talked with my doctors, and explained that this vacation was much needed since I was done with chemo and radiation. All my doctors thought it would be a good idea for me to travel at this time because when August hits, I would not be able to travel for a while. I was so excited!

I called my best friend and told her the news, and she was ecstatic! It was July by then, and I had to get ready for my trip. It was going to be a long car ride. My mom recommended that I take some medicine for my head in case I became nauseous. The chemo and radiation were still working in my body, so I sometimes became ill. My mother and I went to the store and bought more motion sickness bands in case I had issues.

The day of the trip came, and I was all packed and ready. The car ride felt like forever! Of course, we often stopped for bathroom breaks and to tour different towns we drove through. I slept a lot during the trip, but I enjoyed my time as best as I could. Even though I was off chemo, I still had to drink alcohol in moderation. I only had some wine during the trip. We finally arrived in Florida! Her mom and dad rented an Air BNB, where we stayed. It was a beautiful house with a pool. While there, we went to see the fireworks for the Fourth of July with her family. Not only was it beautiful, but it was amazing to be in another environment and to get away. That same day, I prayed and told God, "thank you." "Thank you for allowing me to get away and experience a vacation with friends and family." Even though it was not the cruise I wanted to go on, God let me experience a memory I would never forget.

> **You see, God makes us wait on things, not because He wants us to suffer, but because he has better timing.**

The next day we went to the beach, and feeling the sand hit my feet felt breathtaking. I kept repeating, "Wow, I have my life back." We sat out in the sun and tanned for a while during our time there. While my friend and her family were playing volleyball and exploring the beach, I stayed low-key and relaxed. I knew I could not do that much because I was still weak from the prior treatments I had received. The next day passed, and my friend's mom said, "Let's all go to New Orleans!" In my mind, I was like, "Huh, another trip?" She had mentioned it was only about five hours from where we were. I was ecstatic because I had never been there before. We left Florida the following day and arrived in New Orleans that afternoon. We stayed at a hotel on the strip of Bourbon Street. It was the middle of the week, so many people were outside. Walking in the streets, hearing the bands, and seeing the different vendors outside made me feel like I was in a different world. The evening passed, and the streets were still filled with people and many couples and families exploring. My best friend and I had ventured out that night and had one of the best nights of my life. When we returned to the hotel, I prayed and thanked God again for the experience.

Once I returned from the trip, I was exhausted from all the activities. I had a few weeks to prepare for my extensive surgery. In all honesty, I was not that nervous. I believe God took the anxiety away.

I only had a few more weeks until surgery. I started to have more guests come over. I had friends travel to see me from other states. My grandparents came up from Florida again to help me after the surgery when my mom and brother were at work and school. Many other friends and family took me to my appointments after my grandparents returned home. I felt so loved and touched by those who truly cared and prayed continuously for me; I felt at peace. I started to get invited to places. I was invited to a Sip and Paint event with my cousins. I truly appreciated those moments. It helped get my mind off reality. I was able to run away with my thoughts while painting. There were times when my friends wanted to go out to lounges or bars, and although I could not drink, I substituted liquor for cider which was not bad. I knew that my life was more important than a drink. On days when I was not tired, I would write. I always got lost in my thoughts when writing. Writing was one of my coping skills. Whenever I wanted to vent, writing became my best friend. Some days I asked, "Why me?" Writing was one way that saved me from complaining out loud.

As time passed, I had to let my body rest from chemo and radiation because I had to prepare for my surgery to get my cancer taken out by August 2016. These months were some of the best times of my life. A friend from high school introduced me to an organization I started engaging in. When I had my good days, I would participate in activities, and when there were bad days, I would have someone from the organization tell me about their experience from the event I missed. I met some wonderful people in that organization! We clicked because most of them were battling cancer as well. I remember being invited to walk in a fashion show for cancer survivors. Never would I have thought that I would walk in a fashion show! I have always been called shy. Walking down that runway made me see how strong I really was. It showed me that even though I was sick, I did not have to look or act like I was. I started thinking, "I'm going fight until I can't fight no more."

At this point, I had stopped eating meat, and I had stopped putting sugar in my foods. I did not want my cancer to progress; instead, I wanted to make sure I was doing what I needed to get better. I was receiving treatments at Johns Hopkins, and a social worker insisted that I model in a fashion show they were having in one of the buildings. I accepted the offer. When I went to the event, I met this pretty lady standing in front of a big crowd talking. She was very tall for a female, with gorgeous skin. I remember hearing about her and how she was also diagnosed with the same type of cancer as me, but she was staged at 4. When I met her, she had the purest heart and was quite humble. She had the *badest* catwalk! I started seeing her more and more at events; she always smiled and was energetic. I told myself that if she and all these other people I know going through this horrible illness are smiling and living their lives, then I need to do the same. She gave me hope.

Some time passed, and medical bills started rolling in. It was tough to pay them because I had stopped working. My insurance covered some, but not all. Luckily, I was still old enough to return to my mom's insurance until I turned 26. A friend of mine insisted on making me a Go Fund Me page. I was not too fond of that idea because I did not want people to think I was penniless. I was blessed to meet this young lady because she always gave me words of wisdom to get me through the days. Once she made my account, donations started coming in, and all I could do was shed tears. I did not realize how many people cared that much to give money out of their pockets for me. It helped me remarkably. I was very grateful!

The days seemed to get longer because I was always sitting around. I told myself that I needed to motivate myself and move around. I started doing more with the organization; it felt good being out in the community helping for a great cause. It brings you closer to one when you share the same experience as someone else. I participated in another fashion show. At this point, I thought I was a model! I felt loved when my family and friends would come and watch me. I never really got to do these things when I was in school because I was fearful. This journey made me confident and vigorous.

The night before the surgery to remove my cancer, I packed my bag because I did not know how long I would stay in the hospital to recover. The treatment team explained that I could not eat the day before my surgery and would have to change my diet after the surgery. I was not too thrilled, but I sometimes knew things required sacrifices.

It was surgery day! I had butterflies in my stomach, but I also knew that God would be on time to make me come out stronger. I felt angels surrounding me and giving me all their glory. I was at peace. I knew my mom's thoughts were all over the place. I prayed for her that day because I knew how much she was worried about me. I wanted God to give her strength to get her through that day. I also needed her to be strong for my brother. My younger brother is always to himself and does not like to talk about his feelings much. He is also the most intelligent person that I know. He jokes at the right time and is very talented and dedicated. My brother's faith in everything is always strong. He is literally an Angel. Knowing that people would be hurt since I was about to be in surgery for 10 hours was tough.

As we walked closer to the elevator, it began to get quieter and quieter. We walked in, and there were others in the waiting room that were having surgery as well. The representative asked me for my identification and insurance card. She seemed very lovely, being that she was smiling very hard at me. As I waited for my name to be called, my mom started getting calls from family members. My family was sending me warm thoughts. It was so nice to know that my family was concerned. "Jasmine." The nurse called my name. I was ready; I had already had a long conversation with God. She walked me back to the procedure room and took my vitals. She told my family to wait in the lobby until I was properly set up for my procedure.

Once I changed out of my clothes, my grandparents, family, and friends came back to my room for support. I wanted to tear up because I knew the next road in my life would not be easy. I had to realize that God was testing my faith. My family watched the treatment team take me back to the operating room, and the emotions on their faces broke my heart. It is like I heard a little prayer from every single one of them in my head. I did not know what would happen when guided behind those closed doors. I just knew that God makes no mistakes.

10 hours later. I felt weak, blind, and confused. I was starting to wake up. I wanted to sit up, but I felt numb. It was like something was holding me back from sitting up. I saw an IV in each arm, and my gown had little blood stains everywhere. There was a tube in my nose from which I could barely breathe. There was also a tube that looked like a strong straw on the side of my stomach near my ileostomy bag. You know, I thought I was going to be scared to wear the bag, but I was not. I was more so blessed to wake up and be alive. I felt like a brand-new person! It was like I could see an aurora around me. Something felt new about me that I could not figure out. My mental state was different. I was no longer afraid and felt like I should have been in more pain, but I was not. It was like God took all pain away from me.

As I looked over, my family came in to greet me and tell me that they were so excited to see me awake. I asked how long the surgery took, and someone said, "forever." It did not feel like 10 hours went by, that is for sure. When my grandfather came in, he had his camera. He has always loved cameras and taking pictures. He told me I showed him the ileostomy bag on my stomach. He said I told him to take a picture of it, and he got a kick out of that! I was happy to see him.

After a while, the nurses could take me to my room, where I would stay until I healed. Surprisingly, being there was not lonely. I had plenty of cards and flowers to cherish while I was there. Every day, I had visitors to keep me company while I was going through the healing process. I didn't particularly appreciate how I had to change my diet while at the hospital. The team wanted me to eat fibrous foods since I now had an ileostomy bag. The doctor said that the cancer had been removed, and a biopsy was taken to be analyzed to see whether the cancer got into my lymph nodes. The nutritionist explained the importance of carefully eating because I had just had major surgery. She went on to say that ileostomy bags have certain foods that they can endure.

It was my first night by myself, and my bag started leaking. It happened right when the tech walked in to draw my blood. I was extremely embarrassed. The nurses came into my room to help me get cleaned up. After one night of clean up became two nights, and so forth. I had been at that hospital for almost a week and had an accident every day. My doctor said it was normal and that I should start eating the right foods so my stool could bulk up. I started doing bed exercises every day to help get my muscles working. Getting up to go to the bathroom was a challenge because I could not walk that well. It was like learning how to walk again.

I finally received approval to be discharged from the hospital. It had been a week since my surgery. My doctor said I would have chemo while wearing my ileostomy bag for six months. I was numb to everything. I knew that I did not choose this path but that the path chose me. A few days later, my pathology report confirmed no cancer in my lymph nodes. At that moment, I began to bow and cry out to God!

Time went by, and I started to get my strength back gradually. On my good days, I would write in my journal, pray/meditate, and enjoy the fresh air. I would always ask my brother to go on walks with me, and we would engage in deep talks. I always asked him how his music was coming along. His love for music is his passion. His dedication completes me and makes me want to do better in life. He inspires me to be the best version of myself. God created an Angel when he made my brother; it is like he has been around before. Spending time with my brother throughout this process taught me much about him.

A week passed by, and I started to feel weird. I could not describe the feeling, so I began to lie down because I had no energy. I then realized that I could not urinate. I had been drinking fluids but felt stiff. That evening, my family drove me to the doctor to get evaluated. We were hoping that I did not have any infections from my surgery. The doctor ran tests but did not find anything. She gave me some medicine and sent me home. Since I could not get any answers, I went home, drank a gallon of water, and fell asleep.

A few days later, I received a call from a marketing agent from the hospital. He wanted to put me in touch with a salesperson whose company had a theory on an ileostomy sensor device. The sensor device was to help one know when their bag was full so that it would not overflow and cause accidents. I thought it would be a beneficial tool, especially while asleep. Sometimes I would have accidents in my sleep. I thought, "If my phone could alert me to tell me that I needed to go dump the bag, that would be helpful." The salesperson was very genuine and pleasant. He was passionate about what he did and worked with me to get the device to work. Sometimes, I would meet up with my doctor, and the device would not work correctly, so the doctors were not impressed. I had to report back to him to let him know the news. He had people worldwide working on the device and wanted the product to work. He told me how he appreciated me working with him and that he would always keep me in his prayers.

It was now towards the end of the month, and I started having my down days, but then again, God always gave me helpful resources to get through the day and to find peace. One day I spent the day with my grandparents and uncle, but I felt like I was drowning. I told my nana that I felt lightheaded and could not stand up. My grandparents then took me to the hospital, and come to find out, I was very dehydrated. It was good that I got there in time, or I would have passed out. My nana sat with me and talked while the nurses had me on an IV infusion. That night I went to bed feeling better, but my family wanted me to keep fluids down because I would get dehydrated quickly. The next day came, and I slept for most of it. I woke up feeling weird during the night, and my stomach was in excruciating pain. I tried to go to the bathroom but lost my balance because I was lightheaded. Luckily, my mother heard me before I fell and hit the floor. She immediately called my doctor, and they told her to bring me to the hospital. The pain was unbearable and felt like sharp knives going slowly down my stomach. I felt weak, and I had nothing left in me. The doctor ran tests, and it turned out that I had a life-threatening infection called C Diff (Clostridioides difficile) --inflammation of the bowels.

The next day was rough. I was in pain and felt weak. I told the doctor I wanted to sleep so I would no longer feel the pain. When the doctors were gone, I began to reflect. I literally cried out to God and screamed on the inside. I could not understand why he was giving me all of this. I prayed, "Dear God, please get rid of this," I said that about five times. I said, "His plan is better than mine, and I'm ready to fight through this." Even though I was getting dizzy again, I prayed through it because I knew my God was a healer.

Take the weak thoughts out
of the equation. Yes, we bend,
and we fold, but only God can
postpone. Trust the process, and
he will show you progress.

Self-Reflection

What good came from your struggle? How did you lift yourself up and get through when you were at breaking point?

Self-Reflection

Self-Reflection

Self-Reflection

Self-Reflection

Self-Reflection

Self-Reflection

How Faith Saved My Life

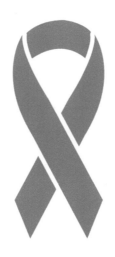

The following day was here, and I felt brand new. I had a little more energy than the previous night. The air even felt better. After I showered and got situated, my doctor came in and said she had some good news for me. She said, "I know how we talked in the past about you receiving a port and IV for chemo; that will no longer happen." She also voiced that I would only take chemo orally. I smiled, she probably thought I should have something more to say, but God knew how grateful I was inside. I went home that night and cried.

> **God, you did it again. You are truly amazing, and I owe you my life, God. You are molding me into the person that you want me to be. You knew all along what the outcome would be, but instead, you tested me. You know how strong I am, and you would never give me anything I can't handle.**

I live by this quote, "I can do all things through Christ who strengthens me." Philippians 4:13 (NKJV)

A few weeks went by, and I started to recover. The medicine that the doctors gave me for my treatment was working. Family and friends continued to visit me, and the new chapter of my life was starting to evolve. The doctor completed my discharge papers, and I could go home.

The following month, I visited my doctor, and we discussed my recovery plan as to whether my ileostomy would be permanent or temporary. If I had to keep it, that would have been fine since I was already used to wearing it. She said that it would be able to come off within the next nine months. After reconstruction, the doctor explained that I should start squeezing my anus after a month to learn to control the bowels. It was good to hear that I could return to my usual self.

Months passed, and I was starting to get used to the bag. People could not tell I had a bag on unless I showed it to them. Most people could not tell that I went through everything I went through. Since I was cancer free and was feeling better, I could leave the house more and engage in activities with my friends and family. I had some bad days because I was still on chemo, but I enjoyed life on my good days. By this time, I had lost 20 to 25 pounds, but I was still eating right to get the protein I needed. Some foods I would try that I used to eat still were tasteless. I was getting used to eating seafood because I stopped eating meat after being diagnosed.

Over time, I started participating in different events associated with cancer. Meeting new people and finding people who went through the same situation helped me tremendously. It was like having a support group. I started sharing my story through poetry at events and posted my experience on social media to help others get through their situation. I spoke to many people each day to give them hope and guidance. I wanted to inspire people and let them know that with God, anything is possible. Pain changed me but made me more cautious of what I was intaking in my body. Pain changes people, and I realized that. Life is too short, and as the saying goes, "Give people their flowers while they're still here, not just while they're sick. "

One day I was driving in the car, and I started listening to my favorite radio station, and the host was giving out tickets to Lupe Fiasco's concert. I was curious because I had never won anything on a radio station before. I called three times, and the line was busy. Something told me to dial one more time, and someone finally picked up! I could not believe it. I had no idea what to say because I did not know if the tickets had been given away already. I said, "Hi, I was calling for the Lupe Fiasco tickets." I am unsure what number caller I was, but he said I won! I was so happy because I had not been to a concert in a while. I loved the feeling of having my life back. The feeling was as if I had won a million dollars. That is how happy I was. I immediately asked my brother if he would attend the concert with me and he said yes. We had a blast, and it allowed me the opportunity to spend quality time with him.

As time went on, I met more of my survivor sisters at a dance workout event. Back then, the Mannequin Challenge was popular, and the group made one. I am unsure if the dance class wore me out, but my stomach started hurting that night I got home. I am also unsure if it was something I ate, but my bag had come off my stomach that night. I thank God I was not out because if so, it would have been a mess. Luckily, I had a strong mindset and did not let the situation set me back. I cleaned myself up, had a glass of water, and went to bed. I was able to go to sleep peacefully.

It was close to December, and I was still out of work. I was starting to apply for jobs because the doctor released me to go back to work. She recommended that I have an office job where I could sit because a lot of moving around would not be beneficial since my energy was still low and I was still on chemo.

A few months after, I stopped participating in the cancer organization. I will not get into why, but I discovered that the money I gave to the organization went elsewhere. The feelings that I went through during this period were challenging. I cried some days and lost sleep at night. Knowing that I looked up to this organization and that it turned out to be a scam was quite upsetting. One night, I was in deep thought and realized that I could not allow the circumstances I faced to get me down. I made great friends that also survived cancer, so I believe I was supposed to cross this path for a reason.

Not long after, I received a call from a manager to interview me to work for the county government. I was so excited because I felt like my life was turning around. I knew I only had a few days left to be on chemo, so I knew I would be ok to work. The manager mentioned that I would work at a desk and do some financial duties. Although my degree was not in finance, I thought of this as a blessing to venture out into something different and get experience in a new career.

I interviewed the next day, and things went well. The following week the manager called me back and told me I had got the job! I cried tears of joy and gave all glory to God. I knew I could get a job, but because of what I went through, I never knew when that day would come.

About a week later, my doctor told me I could stop my chemo pills. She stated, "The time has come, and you are a step closer to being completely done. Now that you are stopping your chemo, you might feel a bit weird for a couple of weeks since you are stopping cold turkey." I felt good when she said that. I felt like everything was falling into place. I just started my new job, and now I would be off chemo. Up next, I would be getting my ileostomy bag taken off! I knew that things would not always be great through the journey, but before I went to sleep that night, I thanked God again for giving me the strength and resources to get through. My prayer went something like this:

God, thank you so much for carrying me through. Thank you for sending me your strength and teaching me what faith really is. My faith really connected me to you. I followed your lead, and with you, I have everything. Thank you for working behind the scenes and pushing me to be uncomfortable. My thought process has truly changed; from this day forward, I will always count my blessings.

Months passed, and I worked for the county government for almost three months. The time was near to have my surgery to remove my ileostomy bag. I was excited but nervous at the same time. The doctors always give you these long speeches about what could possibly go wrong. Sometimes you never know what could happen. I hated hearing about those things, but I understood why they had to inform me.

In a few days, I would have my bag off. I was thinking, "Would my life go back to normal? Would this whole process ever happen again?" I had to get those negative thoughts out of my system and focus on something more positive. My mom had told me she had taken off that day and was excited for me. I had to prepare for my extensive surgery. I had to fast for a day and a half and drink that nasty prep I had in the beginning when I had my first colonoscopy. I told myself, "This time, I am going do what I must do." I could hear my grandmother from Ohio telling me, "Drink it. There is happiness on the other end." The following day, I was ready for my surgery. I was not nervous. I just knew that I would be my old self again when I awoke from surgery. I thought, "am I going to have to learn how to use the bathroom again, or will I miss the bag."

Those negative thoughts in my head disappeared. Once I prayed, I started my prep. This time, the doctors gave me a different prep called MiraLAX. It was not as bad as the last prep that I had. I was able to down the prep with no problems. The following day, the journey ended. My family took me to the hospital, and it was over as soon as the nurses put me to sleep. I woke up in recovery with no problems, and the bag was off. "Thank you, God," I said.

Life is like a long journey that cannot be described. You never know what might come up in your life. You may be excited about going on vacation or getting a new job, but you can never question why God might have taken things from you. Cancer has taught me about myself in so many ways. It made me open my eyes to see how strong I really am. I was so afraid of needles initially and did not want to go through with the process of being healed. I guess God knew I was stronger than I thought I was because I got needles almost daily. He gave me resources through this whole process to get me by. The next thing I knew, my doctor prescribed me a numbing ointment for when I got shots.

I share my story to tell you that life is not easy, but it's not hard either. We are given many resources, but it is up to us whether we use them or not. We all have choices. I had to go through something like this just to really see how strong I really am. I wrote something one day. It said, "We might be uncomfortable or dispirited, but that is only for the moment. That feeling, that pain, it does not last forever. Nothing lasts forever. So, when I am feeling good, I really embrace that feeling. I inhale that energy because tomorrow, that feeling may depart."

> **See, my God knew that I was built for this moment. He knew that I had a message to share.**

I know you may be wondering why I would say that at this moment. Well, because we must fight sometimes, we should be strong and lean on others for comfort and venting. We must realize that every day is not promised. I share my story to bring inspiration to people. I want to save lives. I pray every day, thanking God for saving my life.

I am at peace with myself, and troubles do not worry me as much anymore. I am more spiritual now and have a deeper understanding of what life means. It means to have no worries and to use God as a source. It has drawn me closer to my purpose and helped me understand that my journey will not always be easy but will make me wiser. Now I leave you with some words of encouragement. Be Blessed!

> **I never look at why I do not have something anymore; instead, I focus on being grateful for what I do have.**

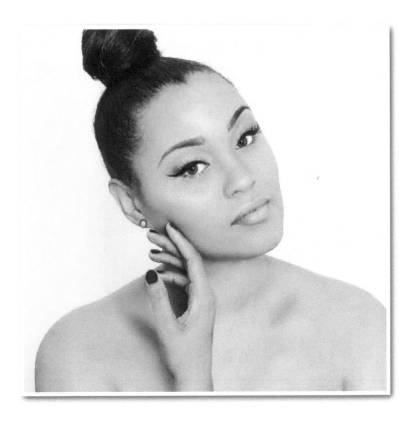

Self-Reflection

Has a point in your life ever changed your perspective? How has an issue you have faced molded you into the person you are today?

Self-Reflection

Self-Reflection

Self-Reflection

Self-Reflection

Self-Reflection

Self-Reflection

Poetry

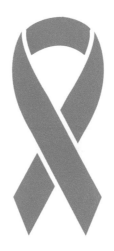

My Pain Converted into Blessings

It is like flowers bloom, and the sun seems
close to the moon.
But things do not seem right on my side because I am
suffering, shifting different ways, paralyzed.
Some days keep thinking I am being used in some ways,
maybe God is using me, preparing me for
this thing called 3.
Yes, stage 3, to be exact. Colon Cancer. I just need some
answers, why me?!
What would you do if you only had 5 years to live?
I was only 23. I have family and friends; this cannot be
happening. I cannot leave!
What if you were told that you would not be able to have
kids and that you would have to freeze your eggs, but
there is a chance that you might not be
able to carry the baby.
I spent hours thinking what did I do wrong, too many
things, I hate my life! I got people leaving left and right.
Cannot even keep this anger outside, knowing I cannot
even hold a baby inside.
I can feel my blood pressure rising, and I am just
beating myself up and slowly dying.

What if you had to take a drug every day that made you
sick to your stomach?
A drug that was made to help you live, but who
knows if it really is...
Chemo brain, chemo mouth, chemo feeling, whatever
the name is, it is not healing...
I wear blue for colon because I am stuck in this bed
glued because the chemo meds got me looking like I am
going through the flu.
Multiple surgeries and needles every day, doctors rush-
ing trying to take this pain away.
This is wrong, spiteful, and hurtful, to the point that I
drop to my knees, asking God, why, please!
Chemo cannot be the key. I am just trying to live happily.
Needles in my side, blood in my eyes, I am getting weak,
and I cannot speak.
That is when I realized, was this all a game? Will I be
able to unbreak this leash? No, because the heat from
the radiation is burning me.
I am not trying *to* scare y'all, I'm trying to inspire all.
Keep your mind right and make you see life
through my eyes.
Because my eyes do not lie, from this pain I feel inside.
Burning sensations, rapid vibrations, burning urination,
frequent movements, bowel movements.
Y'*all* wearing designer clothes with the minks and the
furs while I'm wearing an ileostomy bag on my stomach.
Sitting here comfortable while lying in the hospital bed,
feeling vulnerable.

You trying to get money, but I am trying to survive.
I give my all to be alive!
Many can't even buy this disease; this disease
eats all hope alive.
Takes my heart and crushes it alive, leaving me
hopeless to die.
See now, I am not giving up. He is working behind the
scenes; he knows me better than I know my cancer.
I bow on my knees every night to take my pain away,
and he answers.
My faith saved my life, my pain changed my life. You see,
I knew I was not going to die. I knew I was
going to survive.
I was not going die because I'm a believer in the word,
and only the strong survive.
You see, He said in all things God works for the good of
those who love him. Not cancer but God!
I am a stage three colon cancer believer, thriver, motiva-
tional, inspirational, sensational,
undefeatable survivor.
He is always on time. He saves lives.
He is alive, and He saved mine.

You Saved Me Again

My heart hurts
I can barely swallow
These tubes in me make me feel worse
My energy is gone and I am not the same
Get on my knees everyday just to stay sane
The room is vacant
There is no sound
Treatment team all around me and my mind needs an
escapement
Slowly closing my eyes and drift away
Asking God to take this pain today
Today, tomorrow, and the next
I have future plans
I have a family
I can't leave loved ones behind
Please don't make this a tragedy
Leaning on you for guidance
Slowly drifting back to positive thoughts in silence
Thinking about all of the times you have lifted me up
You will never leave or forsake me
I will keep being strong through it all
I know your will and I am trusting the process until

This is my Truth

I love hard
I worship harder
Life falls apart and I reach out to God
I am a fighter
I let no struggle define me
My thoughts say hold on a little tighter
I seek no acceptance
I am a believer otherwise I am a healer
I believe in giving but not to receive
I stand as one, and over time my life feels like a home
run
I made it, I achieved, should I be displeased?
No, because my experience transformed
Not only am I living confirmation, but I am also an angel
on earth.

Question & Answer

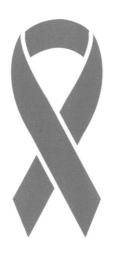

What day were you diagnosed with cancer?

I was diagnosed with Colorectal Cancer Stage 3 on March 2, 2016, and my tumor was removed on August 3, 2016. My ileostomy reversal was on April 24, 2017.

Before your illness, were you familiar with cancer?

I always thought that if someone had cancer, they would not make it. It was a scary feeling when hearing that word. Not many people I knew in my family had cancer until I was diagnosed.

What is your perspective on your diagnosis?

My diagnosis changed my life drastically and saved my life. My perspectives and decisions are different now. I try not to fuss about anything, realize life is precious, and take my time with decision-making. As soon as I stopped worrying, is when I received more blessings. The excuse that I am too young for this had to stop. I would see kids suffering from this disease and even sicker than I was. I would always think, "I should not be complaining when I can still walk and talk!"

I had a little heart-to-heart with myself and told myself that there were some changes I needed to make within myself. I thought, "I'm going do what I have to do to get better, and I am going keep living my life." When people complain, I tell them, "don't complain before God gives you something to complain about." You know, I sit back and think how I was so afraid of needles. Now that I have been through that process, when I go to get my shots, it's easier to handle them now. One day, I started thinking about my purpose on earth. I believe that one thing I am here to do is relay messages. After that experience, I felt reborn. I thought, "Wow, I have never experienced God like this."

How was your experience dealing with cancer at a young age?

I took it one day at a time. Some days I felt like I did not know who to trust. Dating was strenuous because once people saw that I had a bag on, they either disappeared or made an excuse not to communicate anymore. People were cruel some days. I was judged because I didn't look like what I was going through. I used my accessible parking placard when I went into the store one day and when I returned, there was a note on my car window that said, "You are a piece of shit. There are real people in need of handicapped spaces—you suck." I felt low after reading that but remembered that karma is real and to let go and let God.

How were you able to cope with your illness? How was your support system?

My faith kept me going. My family, treatment team, and all my real friends. I say real friends because some people have disappeared from my life. I was devastated. However, I found support by writing my thoughts on paper. It released a lot of emotions. I believe it was better that way because sometimes I had plenty of thoughts on my mind but did not want to talk about them. My family was always by my side entertaining me. My treatment team and real friends were there for me throughout the process, but it is nothing like having someone there who is going through the same thing. Talking to other survivors made life easier because we had much more in common than someone who did not go through the illness.

How has this illness saved your life?

My advice for anyone going through this specific illness would be to try limiting the intake of red meat and highly processed foods and please avoid sugar. *Cancer feeds on sugar.* I realize that everything we do or eat should be in moderation. I started to eat more fruits and vegetables, plus work out occasionally when I had the time. Please take the time to talk to your doctor. Don't think you are ever too young to get a colonoscopy. It is a lifesaver; it saved my life.

How can someone help a loved one who has been diagnosed with cancer?

Be there and comfort them. It does not require much. Sometimes humans just want to have someone's presence around. Several times, I was in the hospital and did not talk much when people visited. I had to be in a mood because I would have good and bad days, but I did appreciate visitors being there even if I did not say much. Someone's comfort and knowing that your love is the best gift anyone could have, especially going through this terrible illness. Never give them the advice you want them to follow; respect their decision. You will run into some who may not want to proceed with treatment. Never judge one's decision. You being there for a person is what helps them to cope. I would say to always keep things normal with a person. Sometimes I felt like my friends were being extra nice and buying me gifts. I do not want to feel like there is something wrong with me. I only want to be treated normally. I have lost many people to cancer, and it truly hurts knowing that they left this world and I was chosen to stay, but I know God makes no mistake

Will the treatment affect you from getting pregnant?

It differs for everyone. I was told that it was a chance I could not get pregnant due to radiation and chemotherapy. It is true. Years later, I discovered my uterus had shrunk, and I would not be able to hold a baby. I also can't have any kids because my fallopian tubes were removed. I always thanked my mom for telling me to go and get my eggs frozen because without going through that procedure, I would have needed a miracle to have kids. I might not be able to have kids on my own, but I have my eggs to allow me to have a surrogate to carry the baby. I realized that God was able to make me see the blessings he gave to me.

Any advice for others going through cancer?

Please take the time to write your thoughts down on paper. Letting your emotions out truly helps relieve stress, which plays a part in self-distraction. I would write letters to myself to help me see my growth throughout the process.

Prayer helped me to stay sane. Everyone has different viewpoints on religion, but I believe I am a child of God, and he is with me every step. Prayer gave me an inner strength that I did not think I had. After praying, I would go into deep meditation and tune out everything around me. This practice gave me a sense of emotional well-being, especially if you are looking for peace.

Helping others with this illness gave me a feeling of joy. It was also a distraction. I enjoyed meeting people and giving some tips I had been learning through the process. Connecting with people with some of the same issues I was going through gave me some relief to know that I was not the only one.

Now that treatment is done, how will your care change?

I meet with my oncologist and surgeon every six months. I get my scans (CT Chest, Abdomen, and Pelvis with IV Contrast) which allows them to see if there are any traces of tumors. A colonoscopy exam is also done, which allows the treatment team to see if there are any changes in my intestine (colon) and rectum. After five years, the doctors explained that I would be released and would need to schedule follow-ups every few years instead of every six months. In all honesty, after my 5-year mark, I will still schedule follow-ups yearly instead of every few years to ensure that I do not have to go through this illness again.

Can you elaborate more on your diet?

Yes! I became a pescatarian immediately once diagnosed. I stay away from meat and poultry but consume seafood. Some foods I eat daily are broccoli, green beans, cabbage, whole grain, baked catfish, baked salmon, baked whitening, little cheese, etc. To avoid accidents, I try to avoid eggs, beans, greasy foods, sugary desserts, etc.

I was always told to eat meat in moderation. I can't say that I followed that rule. I would consume meat daily, so I wanted to make a change and take care of my body the best I could. As stated previously, I changed my diet because colorectal cancer is linked to red meat.

Do you recommend genetic testing?

Yes! This helps you learn if you have illnesses that may run in your family. It may be scary to get the results, but think about it, you can quickly take control over it before it gets out of hand.

What are the signs of Colorectal Cancer?

"In the United States, colorectal cancer is the third leading cause of cancer-related deaths in men and women, and the second most common cause of Cancer deaths when numbers for men and women are combined. (American Cancer Society)" It is also known to be a silent killer. Signs may include pain in your abdomen, blood in stool, bowel habit changes, gas, fatigue, constipation, and weight loss.

Sometimes, people do not experience any symptoms in the early stages. I experienced many of those symptoms because I was at stage 3. It usually depends on the size and location in the intestine.

What made you want to journal your progress?

I knew that it would benefit me one day to look back at all that I had overcome and to measure my growth. I always liked writing phrases or poems to get things off my chest when I did not have the words to share with anyone. Each day I would write down thoughts about how I felt. This coping skill helped me to release a lot of emotion. Who knew releasing emotion on paper would help free my mind. I learned in the end that I fought hard. I faced many challenges that helped me grow and went through experiences that taught me some of the hardest meanings of life.

What is your motivation like now?

I am highly motivated! This journey has taught me never to take anything for granted. I have also learned to work on myself and not seek validation from anyone. I am living for me!

What is your life like now?

Life after cancer has been amazing. I feel like a new person. This process has brought me peace of mind. I became a Pescatarian and am now 30 years old, still living and enjoying every moment. I have a lot to be thankful for. I have been in remission for six years. I get my scans every six months to ensure the illness does not return and colonoscopies yearly. I still have good and bad days and must watch what I eat to avoid having bowel accidents. I had to stop thinking I was sick because if you give in to the fact that you are sick, you will stay sick. I have walked in fashion shows to raise awareness of different types of cancers. I have been featured in articles, tv shows, and many organizations wanting to know more about my testimony.

All those journal entries helped me write this journey of mine. I still face changes in my bowels, such as; loose stool, frequent bowel movements, diarrhea, passing gas, feeling bloated and sore skin around my anus. I will say that I still go through complications with my bowels and have my good and bad days. Unfortunately, I rely on Imodium and some fibrous foods to help get my stool firmer. Imodium helps with watery stools. It starts to slow down my stool, so it takes longer for my stool to pass. I tend to carry a bag with supplies with me each day, such as a change of underwear, wet wipes, a change of clothing, etc., to ensure that I am always prepared on a bad day.

My pain does not define my insecurities, but the path I have crossed defines my maturity.

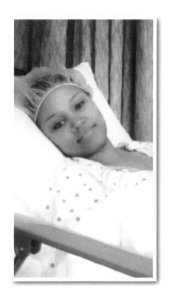
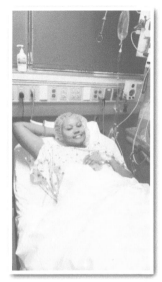

Picture Section:

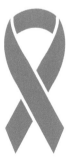

A Trip Down Memory Lane

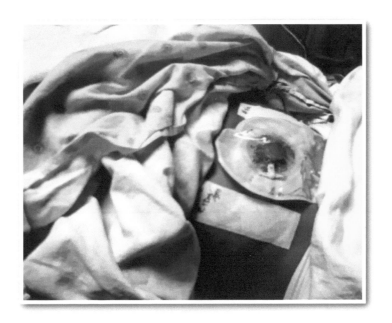

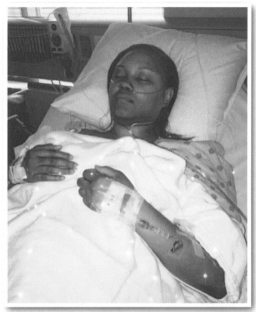

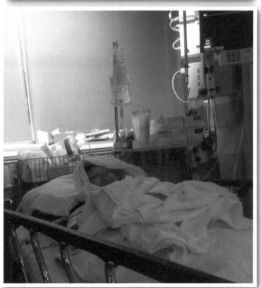

I was still asleep, but it was a successful surgery!

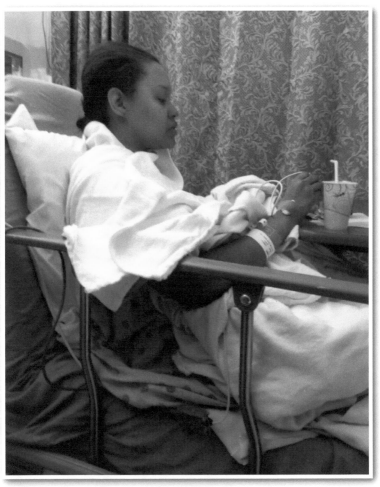

I just woke up from surgery. The nurse gave me a snack to eat and drink.

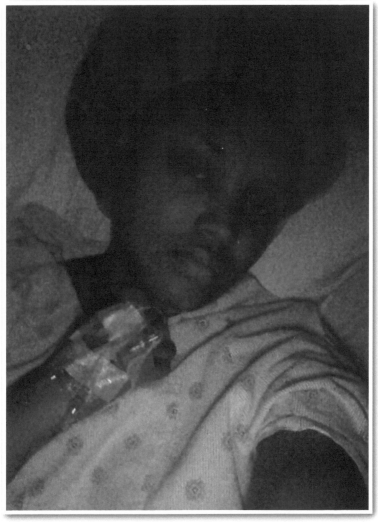

I am strong. I am not afraid of fear. I am a fighter unlocking the door to a brighter day.

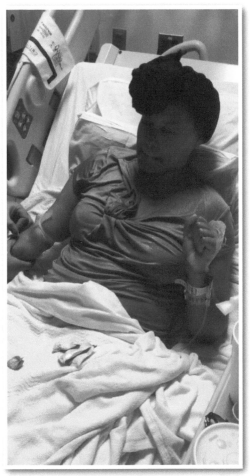

Growth is a series of events. It's not something that is peaceful, it's more of a process. There must be a loss before a win. You must fall before you can walk. You might get some bruises, but all of this is to lead you to your triumphs. Yes, those painful moments were to mold you and prepare you for what's to come. You climb yourself to the top without even realizing it.

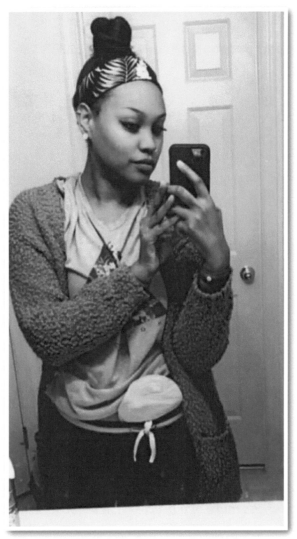

I'm tapping into my soul. I'm realizing who I am becoming. We burn and lose everything just to elevate to greater places.

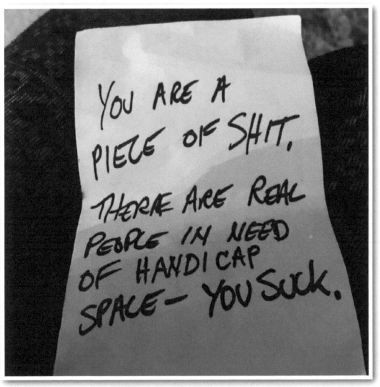

I sit still and let my God handle.

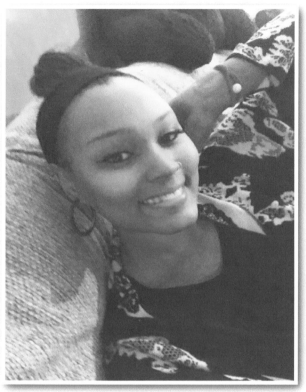

Dear God,

Thank you for blessing me each day and giving me the strength to keep fighting. Day by day things get clearer and I get stronger!

Keep giving me the will to push, to not doubt this process, and to bring me out of the darkness when my mind wonders.

I get to know you more and more as I continue to keep faith. Allow me to understand that this is not the end and continue giving me the resources to understand patience.

Amen.

Jasmine J. Pettross

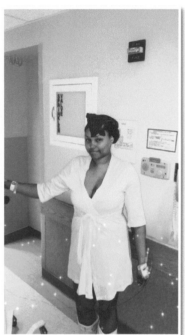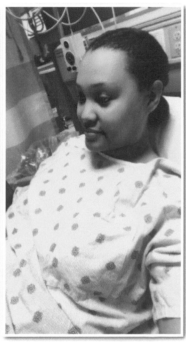

At the hospital recovering from the removal of my ileostomy bag.

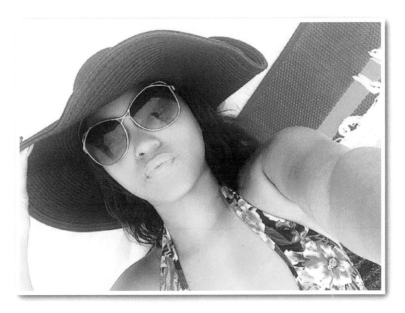

Summer vacation

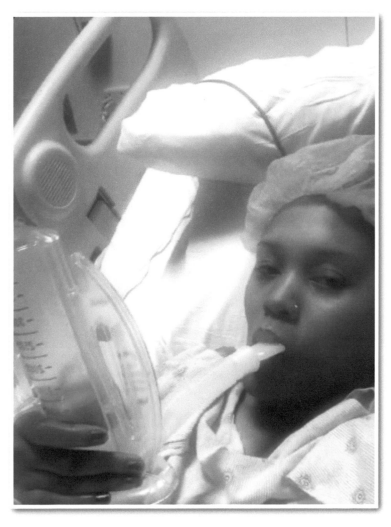

Recovery after surgery.

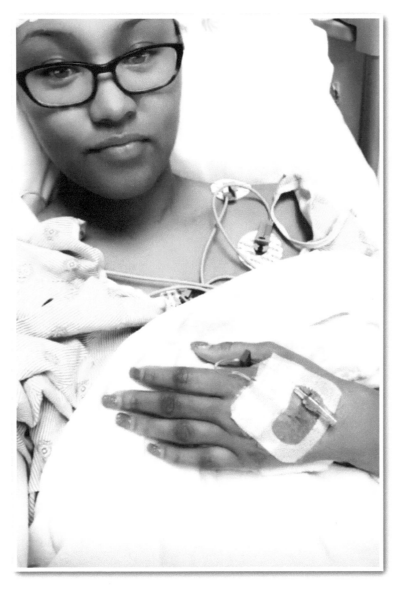

I am still OK.

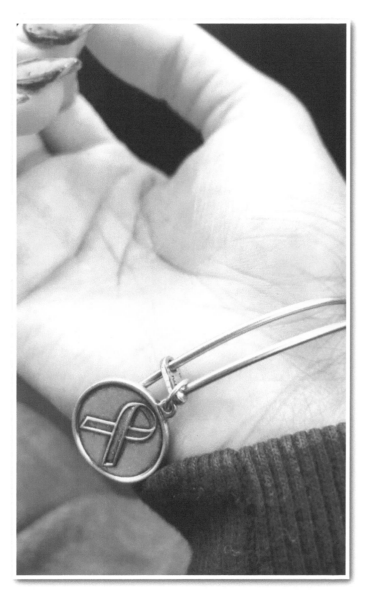

This bracelet represents what I went through.
A friend gave this to me.

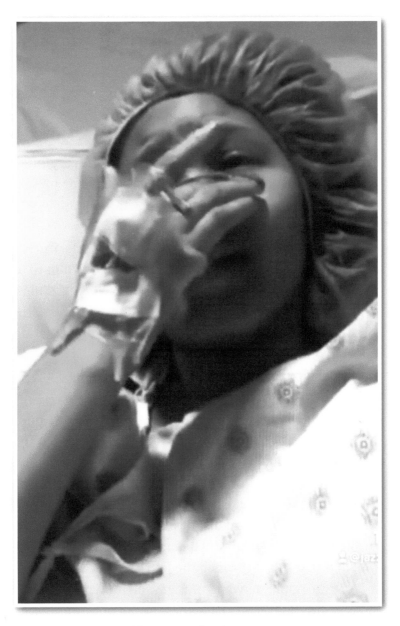

Not every day is easy.

My Testimony

hy me? Hmm. Why not me?

I knew this journey would be heavy, but I always knew God had a reason for everything! The reason was for growth. Perhaps, growth for myself. If it were not for the challenges and overall fight, I would not have the mindset I have today!

I'm not perfect, and we all have flaws, but this process made it hard to love myself sometimes. It made it hard to be a regular person. Once I got into the swing of things, I realized it was time to stop comparing myself to others! I told myself, now is the time to seek no validation from anyone! This is my life, and I have some decisions to make! I realized I had to fight so that I could keep living in my purpose! I had to take time to process my fears and let go of things that were not for me. I started journaling every morning because I was in bed most days. When I could, I would take walks to self-reflect.

I realized that I was special. I was still me, but I was going down a spiritual journey. Once I stopped letting fear in my way and praying, the blessings started rolling in. I had to put myself first! I had no time to lose my mind. I needed that to get through the journey.

At one point, I would put myself down because I thought my body was disgusting because of the marks from the surgery. Throughout this journey, there were times when rude comments were said to me. A person can really start hating themselves because of negativity!

It was hard dating. When people saw my bag, they would disappear. They could not handle it, or maybe they did not want to deal with it. I can actually say thank you to those people. It changed my outlook. I started removing toxic people who were not there for me. I began to become active and help those facing this battle or who may have known someone who had succumbed to it.

I also learned about self-love. Medically and physically cancer hurt but mentally it was a test from God. Self-love takes time, but once you're able to look back and see how far you have come, you will see your worth and be your best you.

Don't give up on yourself. Calculate your progress to see how far you have come and evaluate your improvement. Please be patient with yourself. Find your purpose!

Now is the time to wake up! You may break down or feel unwanted, but you must push! You have to want to change! As long as you are meeting GOD halfway, He will do the rest.

One Year Later– "A Trip Inside of my Mind"

Take time to breathe and self-reflect. I did a lot of this while resting on days I felt weak. I would tune everything out and focus on what I thought a peaceful day would look like. I could see sunny skies and feel a cool breeze while lying on a hammock, rocking back and forth, closing my eyes, and going to a very bright place, thinking about moments I have accomplished and feelings I had when I had hiccups. As I lie rocking back and forth, my mind switches to a time when I was low and felt hopeless. The days that I was alone and did not know what the next day would bring. I realized how throughout this process, I stayed true to myself, laughed, and fought gracefully. Somehow, I always bounced back with a positive attitude.

As I continue to drift in my thoughts, this experience truly made me want to be even kinder than I already am. I have a different mindset about wanting to help others. I received all of these blessings that I now want to give back. Sometimes help is about something other than physically helping someone but recognizing ways to uplift someone. I never thought that my perspective on life would change, but I knew that God always had a plan. I begin to open my eyes and continue to lie in the sun to take all my thoughts in.

I feel that God is preparing me and making me realize the significance and structure of life. Life is unrecognizable. It's a strange storm that makes you weak, punctures you, and motivates you but as you know, storms never last. Once the storm passes, everyone is happy again, feeling sensational and motivated. I am a very deep person, so I see beyond. With each storm, you keep growing, things get clearer, you gain more experience, and you start to get wiser. If you did not fail, you would not be as strong as you are or strong for where you are going. I say all of this: How did your storm make you grow?

Self-Reflection

T ake time to complete this section with aspirations, testimonies, or perhaps storms that made you grow. Reflect on moments in your life that changed your point of view or struggles that made you the person you are today.

Self-Reflection

Self-Reflection

Self-Reflection

Self-Reflection

Self-Reflection

Self-Reflection

Self-Reflection

Self-Reflection

Life After Cancer

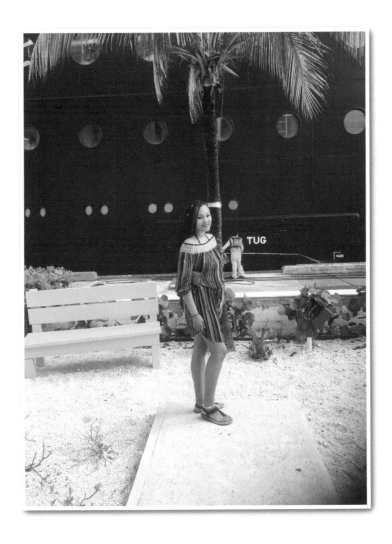

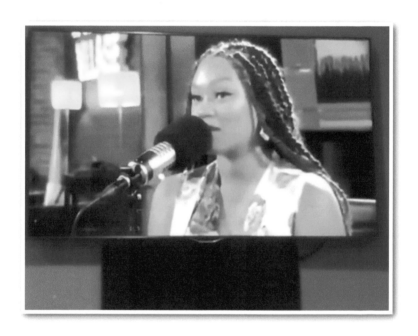

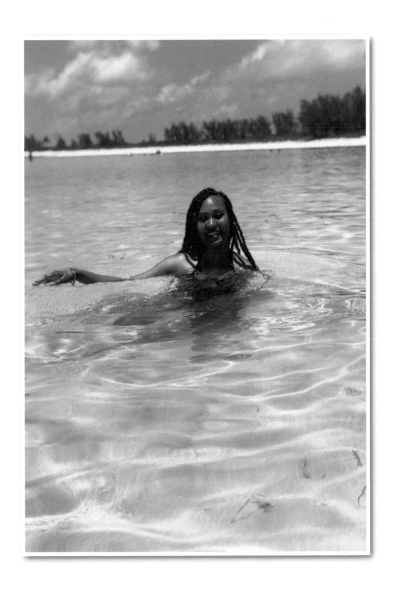

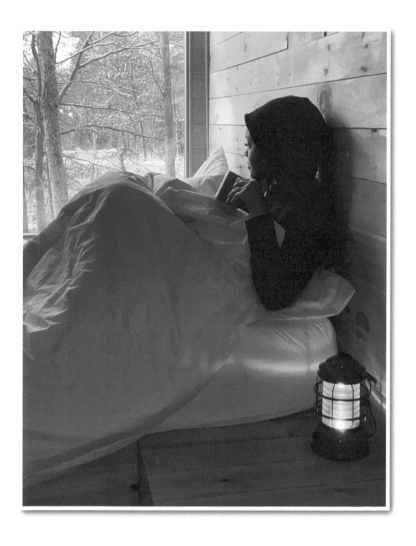

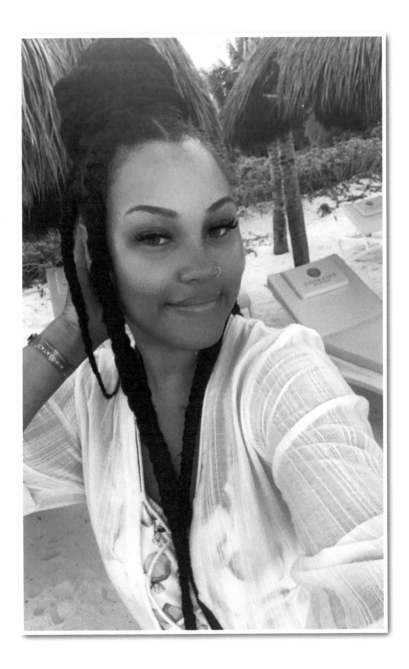

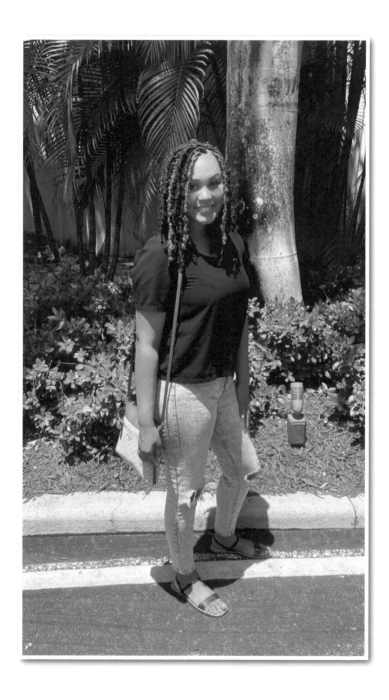

In Loving Memory

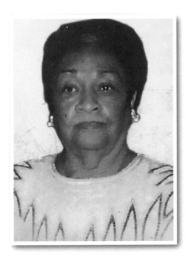

To Estella Jefferson: Nana Ohio, I will always love you and cherish our time on this earth. You were an inspiration in my life and loved me unconditionally. When I was diagnosed, you knew that I would be OK. Your faith in God was so powerful, and you will always be remembered. I love you and always will. Until we meet again, I will always remember what you said, "I want all of you to know that when I'm gone, if I have not told you, just know that I love you, I love you, I love you!"

About the Author

Jasmine Pettross was born in 1992 in Washington, DC, and raised in areas such as Anne Arundel and Prince George's County during her early childhood. She is a cancer survivor, a child of God, and now an author of Faith Defeated My Pain.

Jasmine has an old soul who has received grace and wisdom from her family, whom she loves dearly. On her days off, she loves listening and encouraging people to help them get through cancer. With a major in Human Services, Jasmine graduated in 2014 with a bachelor's degree from Stevenson University in Owings Mills, MD.

As an older sister, she has mastered being a mentor and wants her readers to know that being a survivor comes in all forms. She faced a challenge in her early 20s that sent her a message to convey to her audience that not only did her faith in God allow her to survive, but, He also gifted her with a positive mindset that propelled her to remain alive. Jasmine has been featured in blogs, cancer awareness fashion shows, poetry engagements, articles, podcasts, and segments on TV Shows.

Jasmine is spending her time here on earth to acknowledge her purpose and to help save lives. In her free time, she loves journaling, spending time with family and friends, and traveling.

References

American Cancer Society (n.d.). About Colorectal Cancer. https://www.cancer.org/cancer/colon-rectal-cancer/ about/keystatistics.html#:~:text=Deaths%20from%20 colorectal%20cancer,about%2052%2C550%20 deaths%20during%202023

CPSIA information can be obtained
at www.ICGtesting.com
Printed in the USA
BVHW011334230323
661006BV00001B/1